Parkinson's and the B1 therapy.

Daphne Bryan PhD

Contents

I would like to dedicate this book to the late Dr Antonio Costantini, whose protocol using high doses of thiamine has benefitted thousands. He tirelessly and for no financial reward corresponded with people with Parkinson's around the world, helping them achieve the benefits that he had discovered were possible with thiamine. He was truly an inspired and generous man.

All profits from the sale of this book will go to https://www. gofundme.com/f/high-dose-thiamine-protocol where funds are being raised for future research into B1 for Parkinson's.

Foreword

More than six million people suffer from Parkinson's Disease worldwide, according to recent research[1]. Symptoms of motor and non-motor nature affect their lives and those of their loved ones and to date there is no actual cure for this disease.

When I met the neurologist Dr Costantini in 2010, I had just started my career with the Food and Agriculture Organization of the United Nations in Rome. I was still living in the small town of Viterbo, Italy, commuting to the UN every day by train. Dr Costantini had made a discovery, but needed support to elevate the level of his research and have it published in peer-reviewed medical journals. Like any scientist, I was naturally curious about his initial findings, but not being a Medical Doctor myself, I was particularly cautious about joining him in his endeavour. When I met his first patient in person though, I was instantly hooked. Even my inexperienced and unqualified eyes could not ignore the changes that occurred to this patient's condition as a result of the High Dose Thiamine (HDT) proto-col. Similarly, my mind, and above all my conscience, could not ignore the potential that this therapy offered to millions of patients if even a fraction of them could benefit from this therapy as did the person in front of me on that day. Ever since that moment, when Antonio (Dr. Costantini) explained his theory about HDT and its effects, it became clear to me that this discovery required all of our attention, no matter what it would take.

The next eight or so years have been a whirlwind of strenuous marathons in front of our laptops to submit a manuscript or its revisions on time, swamped in piles of peer-reviewed articles, datasheets with patients' symptoms evaluation scales, and many old school medicine books. In the process we interacted with thousands of patients from all continents, all of them looking for help, ready to give the therapy a try, and to share with us their experiences. We quickly realized we were being pioneers in this research, and with us the patients who willingly decided to support us, to work with us as a team, bonded by a mutual goal and a common objective: to learn to what extent the HDT therapy could relieve others from the symptoms of Parkinson's Disease and to investigate how this could help us understand PD better, to get us a step closer to an actual cure rather than a therapy.

Our small group of scientists had no financial and extremely limited human resources to carry out a gold-standard clinical trial necessary to validate our initial findings and only case reports were manageable for us. As the number of patients increased, we hoped also the number of practitioners and neurologists interested in collaborating with us would have increased, and with it, our chances to make progress in this pursuit. Unfortunately, our wish did not come true, except for one neurologist, Dr. Roberto Fancellu, who joined our team purely based on observations of the otherwise inexplicable improvements of one of his patients.

With Dr Fancellu, we increased our publications, as well as our participation at national and international conferences, presenting our work and calling for support from the scientific community. Although all our interventions have always been well-received, hands abundantly shaken and congratulations profuse, we soon learned that, among the neurological scientific community, collaborative spirit is a featherweight against the fierce competition for success and personal affirmation. We had to look for a way to overcome this problem ourselves.

Once more, with incredible difficulties for a small group of people coming from the Italian province but with the invaluable contribution of patients with PD from the US, we approached the Michael J Fox Foundation in 2019, and submitted a funding proposal for a Phase II clinical trial the following year. Our efforts have been remarkable, though not sufficient to pass the second and last evaluation stage, mainly due to the lack of an infrastructure behind us that could support our hypothesis with the research of potential biomarkers. Or at least, that has been the verdict.

Dr Costantini died in May 2020 leaving us without his leadership and with a void that will not be filled. Although beaten by his loss, we intend to continue his legacy and to seek attention for the potential of his discovery. We created a foundation, the HDT Foundation, to disseminate our work and increase expertise to continue his work, starting with a gofundme campaign (gofundme) to raise funds through a trusted channel for voluntary contributions. All this while still trying our best to support patients who reach out for medical advice.

Finally, when Daphne Bryan wrote to us about the wonderful idea involving this book, we were ecstatic to be able to contribute to its production. This book represents a critical dissemination aid for countless men and women affected by PD who could find solace thanks to the HDT therapy. Our goal, despite the criticism, skepticism and lack of support of the scientific community, is still to carry out a double-blind, placebo-controlled clinical trial on the effectiveness of HDT on symptom control in patients with PD.

Our gratitude goes out to our patients and friends who contributed to the creation of the HDT community of pioneers, through direct contacts and support to us, or through social media and forum groups. Our appreciation cannot be expressed with words but, thank you, anyway.

We hope, through following the pages in this book, that you will learn more about the HDT therapy and find benefits for yourself, or one of the six million people who still suffer every day from Parkinson's Disease. We firmly believe, however, that the scientific community has a duty to follow the lead of our research and the call of so many patients for an unbiased and thorough investigation of thiamine and the symptoms of PD.

Marco Colangeli M.Sc

Scientific Director of the HDT Foundation

---

1. The Lancet, 2018. The burden of Parkinson's disease: a worldwide perspective. Available at The burden of Parkinson's disease: a worldwide perspective - The Lancet Neurology

1. Introduction

It is 200 years since James Parkinson's *Essay on the Shaking Palsy* (Parkinson 1817) was published. In it he describes the characteristic diagnostic features of the condition that came to take his name. Progress on treatment for the condition has, however, been slow and his hopes that a cure, or even a means of slowing down the progression of the disease would be discovered, remains largely elusive.

Parkinson's is a progressive neurodegenerative disorder which is characterized by motor symptoms which include tremor, rigidity, slowness of movement, constipation and balance problems, and non-motor symptoms which include loss of sense of smell, anxiety, depression, apathy, fatigue, pain and sleep problems. The neuropathologic feature of Parkinson's is the degeneration of pigmented dopaminergic neurons in the substantia nigra with the addition of other nuclei (Costantini et al 2015). It has been calculated that by the time a person realises something is wrong, the neuron loss is 68% in the lateral ventral part and 48% in the caudal area of the substantia nigra (Kordower et al 2013). The medication, Levodopa, (brand names include Sinemet and Madopar), has been the gold standard and most effective therapy for Parkinson's for more than fifty years, with alternatives including dopamine agonists, monoamine oxidase B inhibitors and amantadine (Poewe et al 2010). None of these drugs, however, repair or limit the damage caused by the disease, nor do they stop its progression. Furthermore, levodopa can lead to side effects, such as dyskinesia, which can be more troublesome than the original symptoms levodopa was taken to relieve. But what if there was a simple, inexpensive, easily available vitamin which could significantly improve symptoms as well as slow down disease?

This book aims to describe a therapy which uses high doses of thiamine (vitamin B1). It is available to all with Parkinson's, whatever stage has been reached, and was devised and used successfully by an Italian neurologist with his patients from 2011. But before I discuss the science, theories, and research behind the therapy and what the therapy involves, I will explain who I am, why I am writing this book and my own experience with the therapy.

My Story

I am not a medical practitioner. I am a person with Parkinson's who, for the last four and a half years, has successfully used High Dose Thiamine to hugely improve my health. The aim of this book is to bring together all the information currently available on the therapy and present it clearly, so that a person with

Parkinson's, with the support of his/her doctor, will be able to adopt the therapy themselves. The information, used in this book to discuss the therapy, is taken from three areas of resource. Primarily I will report the advice given by Dr Costantini, the neurologist who devised and used this therapy with his Parkinson's patients. I will also add to this relevant information available from other doctors and nutritionists who use high doses of thiamine with their patients to resolve various health issues. Finally, I will include anecdotal accounts from a large international group of people who use the therapy to treat their Parkinson's.

My story, as it relates to this therapy, began in 2017, when a friend sent me an article about the Italian neurologist, Dr Antonio Costantini, who was treating his Parkinson's patients with very high doses of vitamin B1 (also known as thiamine) and seeing their symptoms improve by up to 70%. The article also noted that in the five years he had treated his patients with B1, their illness had not progressed. I had been diagnosed with Parkinson's seven years earlier and was keen to do all I could to slow its progression and so, when I next had an appointment with my doctor and my neurologist, I discussed the therapy with them. Although they had not been aware of High Dose Thiamine being used for Parkinson's, they knew of its use in treating recovering alcoholics and were quite happy for me to take B1, so I purchased some tablets. I was not expecting a miracle. If anything, I felt the story almost too good to be true, so I added B1 to my supplement pile and went about my daily routine not thinking too much about it.

The first of my symptoms to improve was fatigue. Actually, I did not notice that this had happened and only realised I must have more energy when I was telling a friend about all the new hobbies I had taken up. My life, because of the fatigue which often accompanies Parkinson's, had become rather restricted, but after beginning B1, I began training a choir, teaching the piano, learning Italian and watercolour painting!

I did not notice the next symptom relief either. I had been having massages for several years and, at one appointment, my therapist remarked that he noticed a new softness and elasticity in the muscles and soft tissue of my body. Most people diagnosed with Parkinson's find their muscles become more rigid. They might start to hold their neck and shoulders stiffly, lose expression in their face, and find it more difficult to swing their arms as they walk. Two years earlier, I had managed to break the humerus bone at the top of my arm, merely by slipping and jerking my shoulder awkwardly, such was the tension through my muscles. After my therapist had remarked on the change, friends too started telling me how much quicker and more fluid I was moving. One friend noted that I was now smiling "right up to my eyes", yet I had been unaware of the change. I think I had not noticed that my symptoms were easing because, when a movement is difficult, you concentrate on coping with making the movement, whereas when a movement is easy, you focus on the end goal of the movement and do not pay any attention to your good or bad motor skills.

My anxiety and depression lifted too, and my sense of smell improved. However, these symptom changes were very gradual, probably unfolding slowly over three to six months. At the time of writing this, I have been taking B1 for four and a half years. I have seen many symptoms disappear and have seen no real progression of the disease. But how am I sure that it was the B1 which caused these improvements?

Firstly, in my case, I had made no other changes to my protocol. I did not increase my levodopa medication, neither did I add any other supplements during this time. As the B1 was the only change I had made, it is very likely that B1 had caused the improvements. Moreover, when I stopped the B1 for a while, symptoms, particularly fatigue, returned after a few days. Furthermore, I believe B1 was responsible for the changes in my Parkinson's because of the type of improvements that happened. Dr Costantini noted that non-motor symptoms, such as fatigue, loss of sense of smell, poor sleep, gut problems and pain "are often relieved completely by High Dose Thiamine, whereas to date, no other therapy has demonstrated similar effectiveness against non-motor symptoms." (www.highdosethi amine.org) But who was the neurologist Dr Costantini?

Dr Antonio Costantini

Dr Antonio Costantini worked in Viterbo, Italy. By the time I first read about him, he was treating over 2,700 patients with thiamine, (some as face-to-face patients, some via email), using the therapy as an adjunctive treatment to the patients' standard Parkinson's medication. During the five or more years he had been treating these patients, he had noted no apparent disease progression, while symptom improvement had been significant. He published his first study on High Dose Thiamine for Parkinson's in 2013 and published a longer study with other co-authors in 2015. As well as improving symptoms, his High Dose Thiamine therapy also reduced such side effects as dyskinesia, which is often experienced when taking traditional drugs. But he did not only use High Dose Thiamine with his Parkinson's patients. He had been working with the therapy for various health problems since 2010 and published studies on the use of thiamine for Fibromyalgia (Costantini et al 2013 E), Essential Tremor (Costantini et al 2018 B), Spinocerebellar Ataxia Type 2 (Costantini et al 2013 A), Hashimoto's thyroiditis (Costantini et al 2014 B), Multiple Sclerosis (Costantini et al 2013 C), Cluster Headache (Costantini et al 2018 A) and many more.

As well as working with his face-to-face patients in Italy, Dr Costantini very generously gave of his time to personally advise hundreds of people with Parkinson's around the world, via email, and free of charge. Sadly, this came to an abrupt end when he suffered a post-surgery stroke several years ago and while still recovering from this, he contracted COVID-19, and in May 2020, this claimed his life.

Why has my doctor not heard of this therapy?

If you are new to the idea that a simple vitamin could improve symptoms where medication has failed, you may now be asking - Why has my doctor not told me about this? The answer is probably two-fold. Firstly, doctors are highly trained in finding drug and surgery solutions to health issues, whereas nutrition is a very small part of their training. Secondly, to have a novel treatment accepted by the medical profession, it is necessary to produce a rigorous, double-blind, placebo-controlled, multi-based study supporting the hypothesis. There are peer reviewed, published studies available on the High Dose Thiamine therapy but they are either pilot studies or case studies. Dr Costantini's colleagues have planned a large, double-blind, placebo-controlled study but have so far been unsuccessful in getting the funding necessary to carry it out. It is sad to think that there are huge numbers of people with Parkinson's all round the world, who are struggling with life restricting symptoms, who, if put on the vitamin B1 protocol, might be able to enjoy an easier life. I must add here that the Italian team have a 'Go Fund Me' page on the website. If anyone wishes to donate to their planned research project, please go to gofundme

This chapter has merely introduced the therapy. I do not expect my personal story alone to convince anyone that High Dose Thiamine is a therapy worth trying. Chapter 2 will look at the broader evidence for the success of thiamine and present the published research which has studied the effect of thiamine on Parkinson's patients. Their authors' theories as to what physiological effect high doses of thiamine might be having on Parkinson's patients will be presented. The aim of Chapter 3 is to explain clearly how to adopt the therapy, and Chapter 4 will include personal accounts from people who have found that High Dose Thiamine has reduced their symptoms and, as some comment, 'given them their lives back'.

2. The Science

The aim of this chapter is to explore the science behind the High Dose Thiamine (HDT) therapy, to understand what vitamins are, their effect on the body and the effect of B1 (thiamine) in particular. We will consider how thiamine is used in this therapy, its safety and the theories behind its positive effect on people with Parkinson's. Finally, discussion will consider the findings of several research studies which have tested the therapy with Parkinson's patients.

What is thiamine?

Thiamine is the first of the B vitamins. It was first isolated in 1926 and synthesized in 1936. A vitamin is an organic compound which an organism needs in small quantities for normal cell function, growth, and development. Essential nutrients cannot be synthesized in the body, either at all or not in sufficient quantities and therefore must be obtained through the diet. There are 13 essential vitamins. Vitamins A, C, D, E, K, and the B vitamins (thiamine B1, riboflavin B2, niacin B3, pantothenic acid B5, B6, biotin B7, folate B9 and B12). The B vitamins, a group of eight essential nutrients, are needed to help the body convert food into energy, which is known as metabolism. B vitamins also create new blood cells and maintain healthy skin cells, brain cells and other body tissues. Together they are referred to as vitamin B complex.

Not just correcting a deficiency

The High Dose Thiamine therapy uses doses far in excess of those needed to correct a deficiency. Dr Derrick Lonsdale, a specialist in nutrient-based therapies and writer of over 100 published papers, many on High Dose Thiamine, points out that using a vitamin in large doses turns it into a drug (Lonsdale 2021). The daily recommended requirement of thiamine for a healthy individual is just 1.1 mg for women and 1.2 mg for men (www.mayoclinic.org). Even for a thiamine deficiency, the suggested daily dosage is only between 5 mg and 30 mg (www.medlineplus.gov). However, the therapeutic dose used in Dr Costantini's B1 protocol for Parkinson's can be as much as 4,000 mg oral dose per day. Just addressing a deficiency does not explain the remarkable symptom improvement that is seen when high doses of thiamine are used. If the therapy is not correcting a deficiency, what exactly is the high dose of B1 doing?

It is thought that high doses of thiamine can influence cellular energy metabolism which has been disrupted or inhibited by other factors. Cells need energy to work efficiently. The theory of this therapy is that by using high doses of thiamine, certain enzymes involved in energy metabolism are stimulated and metabolic function in the cells is restored, enabling them to work efficiently once more. (Elliot Overton. YouTube - 'Mega-Dose Thiamine: Benefits beyond addressing deficiency'). Enzymes are a type of protein that the body uses as a catalyst to speed up the rate of biochemical reactions. They are responsible for driving the reactions involved in practically every known function of the human body. Vitamins and minerals act as helpers for specific enzymes to work as they should ('Nutrition and Functional Medicine'. Elliot Overton www.eonutrition.co.uk).

Dr Costantini's interest in High Dose Thiamine began in 2011, when he treated a man with spinocerebellar ataxia type 2. Following high doses of thiamine by injection, the man's fatigue and motor symptoms improved. From this, Dr Costantini formulated the hypothesis that in some inherited and degenerative diseases of the nervous system, symptom development could be linked to a thiamine deficiency in a particular area or areas. He suggested that this was either due to a dysfunction of the intracellular transport of thiamine or to structural enzymatic abnormalities. This dysfunction, he thought, could be responsive to high doses of thiamine (Costantini et al 2013). Costantini went on to publish a number of human clinical trials using high doses of thiamine for various health issues. These include spinocerebellar ataxia type 2 (Costantini et al 2013 A), Friedreich's ataxia (Costantini et al 2013 B and Costantini et al 2016 C), fatigue in Multiple Sclerosis (Costantini et al 2013 C), inflammatory bowel disease (Costntini et al 2013 D), fatigue after stroke (Costantini et al 2014 A), Hashimoto's thyroiditis (Costantini et al 2014 B), dystonia (Costantini et al 2016 A), myotonic dystrophy type 1 (Costantini et al 2016 B), chronic cluster headache (Costantini et al 2018 A), essential tremor (Costantini et al 2018 B) and Parkinson's disease (Costantini et al 2013, Costantini et al 2015)

The link between PD and thiamine

Several studies have presented factors which may link thiamine to Parkinson's, to dopamine, and to neurological conditions (Lu'o'ng & Nguyen 2012). Thiamine is a cofactor of enzymes involved in fundamental pathways of energetic cell metabolism (transketolase, alpha-keto-acid decarboxylase, pyruvate dehydrogenase, alpha-keto-glutarate dehydrogenase) (Costantini et al 2015). Mizuno et al (1994) reported a decreased activity of thiamine diphosphate-dependent enzymes in the nigral neurons of patients with Parkinson's. Lu'o'ng and Nguyen (2013) noted several studies which show a relationship between dopamine and thiamine. One study looked at rats, which had been given a thiamine deficient diet, causing them to develop rat-killing aggression. When they were given dopamine, the aggression caused by thiamine deficiency was suppressed (Onodera 1987). Parkinson's patients who take levodopa medication, show significantly higher cerebrospinal fluid levels of thiamine diphosphate and total thiamine than do patients who are not treated with this drug (Jiminez-Jiminez et al 1999), showing a further link between thiamine and dopamine. Sjoquist et al (1988) reported that a thiamine deficiency was seen to decrease the concentration of dopamine in the striatum, a nucleus in the basal ganglia. Gold et al (1998) noted that 70% of their Parkinson's patients had low plasma thiamine and 33% had low red blood cell thiamine levels, showing a further relationship between thiamine and Parkinson's Disease. Finally, Merkin-

Zaborsky et al (2001) successfully treated nine patients, presenting with acute neurological disorders, with thiamine.

Published research articles

There are three studies which have looked specifically at the effect of a High Dose Thiamine regime on people with Parkinson's. An American study by Lu'o'ng and Nguyen (2012) is a preliminary report on five case studies looking at the effect of High Dose Thiamine on people with Parkinson's. Dr Costantini and colleagues, in Italy, are the authors of two further published articles. The first (Costantini et al 2013) reports the effect of High Dose Thiamine on three people with Parkinson's. The second (Costantini et al 2015) is a much larger and longer study, following the effect of the therapy on 50 people with Parkinson's, over a duration period ranging between 95 and 831 days.

Lu'o'ng and Nguyen's case studies (2012) followed five male Parkinson's patients aged between 65 and 82 years old who had been diagnosed between 3 and 16 years earlier. They presented with similar symptoms: mask-like face, infrequent blinking, tremor, Parkinsonian gait with reduced arm swing and occasional freezing and bradykinesia (slowness of movement). The patient in case 4 also had difficulty pronouncing words with constant dribbling and the patient in case 3, a 68 year-old, showed some memory loss. Each patient was given injections of thiamine daily. For cases 1 and 5, the dosage was 100 mg of thiamine injection daily, while for cases 2, 3 and 4, this was 200 mg of thiamine injection daily. There is no explanation as to why the different dosages were chosen. It did not appear to relate to their pre-trial thiamine levels as case 1 had the lowest, suggesting the greater need, but was in fact given the lower injection dosage. Neither did it seem to relate to the length of time since their diagnosis, as case 5 had been diagnosed the longest yet was given the lower dosage.

On the fourth day of the trial, the five participants were observed once more and showed very significant improvements. All had reduced facial rigidity and were reported as 'smiling'. Their walking had improved with longer strides and more arm swing. Tremors also appear to have reduced in every case. It is a little disappointing that the researchers have restricted themselves to observable motor symptoms to gauge for change and have not commented on possible non-motor symptom changes like fatigue, anxiety, brain fog, apathy, sleep etc, which we now know are sometimes early signs of a positive B1 effect. After ten days, cases 2, 3 and 4 were taken off their regular Parkinson's levodopa medication 'without any effect on their movement'. Case 1 and 5 were lost from further study follow-ups.

Although this study clearly shows that Parkinson's patients can react very favourably to high doses of thiamine in a very short space of time, it raises more questions than it answers. Unfortunately, it was a very short study, with no information on what happened to cases 2, 3 and 4 after the ten-day follow-up or whether they continued with daily 200 mg thiamine injections. In their research, Lu'o'ng and Nguven had administered a considerably higher dose than Costantini and colleagues used in their research (2013, 2015). Costantini noted, and personal experience has shown me, that if the dose given is too high for an individual, symptoms can worsen. Did the patients in this study avoid this? Finally, for how long did the three participants, who were taken off their Parkinson's drugs, continue successfully without medication?

Costantini and his colleagues worked in Viterbo, Italy and their case reports (2013) dealt with three newly diagnosed Parkinson's patients not yet on Parkinson's medication, two females and one male aged between 74 and 79 years of age. The patients were assessed first using the Unified Parkinson's Disease Rating Scale (UPDRS). One patient was also evaluated with the Fatigue Severity Scale (FSS). They each presented with bradykinesia, rigidity, mask-like face with infrequent blinking, lack of arm swing when walking, and continuous resting tremor. Their total plasmatic thiamine was tested and found to be within the healthy reference range. Each patient was prescribed 100 mg of thiamine parenterally (by injection) twice a week. This is substantially less than the daily dosage used by Lu'o'ng and Nguyen. Costantini's patients were also given a small dose of group B vitamins at the same time as their B1 injections. After 15 days the three participants were re-examined.

All three now showed normal muscular tone, with a reduction in resting tremor and increase in arm swing while walking. Their UPDRS scores revealed considerable symptom improvements. Case 3's fatigue regressed almost completely. Costantini concluded that the symptoms of Parkinson's are the manifestation of a thiamine deficiency likely due to a dysfunction of the active transport of thiamine inside the cells or due to structural enzymatic abnormalities. He believed that thiamine injections may play an important role in restoring survivor neurons and in limiting the progression of the disease because the dysfunction of thiamine-dependent processes could be a primary pathogenic pathway leading to the demise of dopaminergic and non-dopaminergic neurons in Parkinson's (Costantini et al 2013, Jhala and Hazell 2011).

Costantini and his colleagues mention three 'learning points'. Firstly, that the treatment is immediately available. Secondly, that there is no study in the literature that has observed side-effects linked to the daily use of high doses of thiamine. And thirdly, that their case report opens a ray of hope for therapy of Parkinson's.

The 2013 research by Costantini and colleagues only followed the three case studies for 15 days. Their 2015 research sought to provide a larger and longer study. Fifty patients with Parkinson's were recruited, 33 men and 17 women. Their average age was 70 years and their average disease duration was seven years. Seven of the patients were not yet taking Parkinson's drugs. They were all assessed at the outset using the Unified Parkinson's Disease Rating Scale (UPDRS) and the Fatigue Severity Scale (FSS). They were then treated with 100 mg of thiamine administered by intramuscular injection twice a week without any changes to their Parkinson's medication or personal therapy. All the patients were re-evaluated after one month and then every 3 months during treatment. The follow-up period lasted between 95 and 831 days.

Treatment with thiamine injections led to significant improvements in motor symptoms among the fifty participants. This did not differ between male and female, younger and older, or those on Parkinson's medications and those who were not. Disease duration did make a difference in that those who had had Parkinson's for longer improved comparatively more than the newly diagnosed. Those participants who had reported fatigue before thiamine treatment had found that their energy levels improved significantly. The three patients with clear symptoms of dementia at baseline showed improved cognitive scores at follow-up. The patients improved over the course of about three months and then sustained that level of improvement for the balance of the study. None of the patients on levodopa medication needed to increase their levodopa dosage during the study and those who were not on Parkinson's medications at the start of the trial did not need to start it. None of the patients experienced adverse effects from taking thiamine or needed to discontinue treatment.

Costantini pointed to limitations in his 2015 study, the absence of a placebo-controlled element being the most relevant, though the clinical improvements observed in his patients had been continuous and stable for a long period of follow-up, which does not suggest placebo effect. He also made a point of introducing thiamine therapy to his patients without giving them any information about possible outcome. Furthermore, he tried to avoid the issue of selection bias by including all consecutive patients with Parkinson's who visited his department, without selection.

For Costantini, High Dose Thiamine was an adjunct therapy to be used together with Parkinson's medications if the patient had started them. He did not attempt to take his patients off their levodopa medication during the study, even though they were showing very significant improvements in symptoms. Unlike Lu'o'ng and Nguyen (2012), Costantini did not present thiamine as a cure and believed that drugs like levodopa still had an important part to play in the patient's total therapy. He felt that High Dose Thiamine alone was not capable of leading to a complete regression of motor symptoms unless the disease had had a very recent onset. This, he felt, might be because, even though thiamine restores survived cells and seems to stop the development of the disease, the cells left untouched by the aggression of the disease were in limited number and were not capable of substituting all functional systems that depend on a healthy substantia nigra (www.highdosethiamine.org).

Both Lu'o'ng and Nguyen (2012) and Costantini et al (2013, 2015) gave their patients 'parenteral thiamine', meaning the dose was administered by injection. Lu'o'ng and Nguyen cite several studies which suggest that intestinal absorption of thiamine, used when taking B1 orally, could be impaired. Pfeiffer (2003) says that gastrointestinal dysfunction is common in Parkinson's patients and can potentially affect the therapeutic intervention. Baum and Iber (1984) suggests that although intestinal absorption of thiamine is sufficient in young people, it may be reduced with age. Baker et al (1980) demonstrated that only the intramuscular administration of thiamine was able to correct thiamine deficiencies in subjects over the age of 60. As will be seen in the next two chapters, oral administration of thiamine is both recommended and largely successful in many cases where an injection is not available, but the dosage needs to be high enough to cope with the gastrointestinal absorption problems.

The theories

Costantini and his colleagues (2015) suggested that "the improvement of the energetic metabolism of the survivor neurons in the substantia nigra, due to the high doses of thiamine, could lead to increased synthesis and release of the endogenous dopamine, increased activity of thiamine-dependent enzymes, or better utilization of exogenous levodopa." There was no blood thiamine deficiency at baseline and the fact that high doses of thiamine had such a positive effect on symptoms led Costantini to suggest that Parkinson's symptoms are the result of neuronal thiamine deficiency, probably due to dysfunction of the active intracellular transport of thiamine or to structural enzymatic abnormalities.

Furthermore, there is an interesting connection between thiamine and alpha-synuclein. Mutations in alpha-synuclein are associated with early-onset familial Parkinson's disease and the protein aggregates abnormally in Parkinson's disease, Lewy body disease and other neurogenerative diseases (Goedert 2001). A study into thiamine's effect on alpha-synuclein suggested that an increase of intracellular thiamine could reduce alpha-synuclein concentration and then alpha-synuclein aggregation (Brandis et al 2006).

Side Effects

Costantini reported that among more than 2,500 patients treated with intramuscular injections of thiamine, he only had four allergic reactions (www.highdosethiamine.org). In Costantini and Pala's study of High Dose Thiamine to treat patients with ulcerated colitis and Crohn's disease (2013 D), one patient reported mild tachycardia, which was resolved by reducing the dose. Some patients reported insomnia, which was resolved by administering the last dose by 5 pm. No side effects were reported in the case studies on Fibromyalgia (Costantini et al 2013 E) and Multiple Sclerosis (Costantini et al 2013 D). In their 2015 study on the use of High Dose Thiamine with Parkinson's patients, Costantini and colleagues reported "No patients experienced adverse events or discontinued treatment, the only clinical issue to monitor in patients with diabetes treated with insulin was the slight increase of glycemia levels and subsequent increased insulin dosage." Bager et al (2021), in their trial of thiamine with patients with IBD fatigue, found only mild side effects. "Because thiamine is a water-soluble vitamin with renal clearance, the risk of thiamine accumulation is limited for patients with normal kidney function."

It is indisputable that thiamine has, as demonstrated in these albeit limited studies, a significant effect on the symptoms of people with Parkinson's. Dr Costantini, who treated about 4,000 patients in all, was continually asked by them why other neurologists did not know or were not interested in the thiamine therapy. He invariably replied that he did not know. Official science still says that non-motor symptoms in Parkinson's are untreatable, while Dr Costantini said that they were more sensitive than motor symptoms to HDT treatment. This therapy is not a cure. In none of Costantini's literature does he suggest that it is. To the man or woman with Parkinson's disease, however, it offers the chance to live in an improved physical and psychological condition previously unthinkable.

Dr Derrick Lonsdale, a thiamine expert, wrote (2021)

"The use of a vitamin in mega-doses to treat disease is brand new. It seems that enough clinical evidence of its benign, non-toxic effect has been reported by this Italian group to "set the world of medicine on fire". The concept of using a molecule, essential to life, in large doses as a drug will undoubtedly require further confirmation, but it would be absurd to ignore these results."

Looking to the future

I will conclude this chapter with the words of Costantini's colleagues; Dr Roberto Fancellu (Neurologist), Dr Marco Colangeli (Environmental Scientist), and Ms Maria I Pala (Nurse), who are searching for funding to carry out a full study.

"So many people could benefit from this therapy today. But for every patient in the world to receive High Dose Thiamine therapy through trusted medical channels, it must be approved by various international drug administrations such as the US Food and Drug Administration (FDA) and the European Medicines Agency (EMA).

"Only successful results from a well-designed clinical trial will satisfy the approval process. Specifically, we must conduct a multi-location, randomized, double-blind, placebo-controlled trial covering a representative number of patients and spanning the relevant time frame. Such research requires adequate funding, sustained for the trial duration.

"Discovering suitable sources of possible funding and submitting applications to them demand constant focus and effort. But we must take up the challenge, because successful results from a robust clinical trial would confirm the effectiveness of the therapy scientifically and with statistical significance, allow us to understand and describe its mechanisms, and potentially show us how to further improve its efficacy

"To this end, we launched a gofundme campaign with the ultimate goal of raising funds to move HDT therapy forward into the approval process, and to make information about our experiences so far directly available to patients, practitioners, and other health professionals." (www.highdosethiamine.org).

This chapter has shown that in the currently somewhat limited research, thiamine has been shown to have a very significant positive effect on the symptoms of Parkinson's disease. What is more, the High Dose Thiamine therapy is immediately available, inexpensive and safe. While there is currently no treatment available which will slow the progression of Parkinson's or improve symptoms safely, this therapy has a lot to offer and there is an urgent need for a thorough, research project to explore the therapy's efficacy and fine tune its adoption and use. Parkinson's is a degenerative disease. There is a sense of urgency for neurologists, doctors and Parkinson's nurses to acquaint themselves with this therapy and offer their patients the chance of trying this therapy which for many, could give a substantially improved life.

3. The Protocol

This chapter will aim to explain the protocol of the High Dose Thiamine therapy as we currently understand it. It can, however, only be guidance. This is not a one-size-fits-all therapy. Patients will need to play an active role in deciding which dosage is right for them. It will require some trial-and-error testing as well as patience. The possible improvements, however, when the right dosage is found, are quite substantial to the person with Parkinson's, and should make it well worth the effort.

Although in this chapter I will address people with Parkinson's directly, I recommend that you work with a health professional who is experienced in and knowledgeable about the therapy, if possible. Where this is not possible, at least discuss your desire to try the therapy with your doctor.

What form of thiamine to use?

Three forms of thiamine are dealt with in this book: intramuscular injections, oral (thiamine hydrochloride) tablets, capsules or powder, and sublingual (applied under the tongue) thiamine mononitrate tablets. Each offers advantages and disadvantages of usage, and all can produce good results when a person's 'correct' dose is found.

There are other derivatives of thiamine on the market. Benfotiamine is fat-soluble. Dr Lonsdale, however, points out on his website (https://www.hormonesmatter.com/navigating-thiamine-supplements/) that one published report suggests benfotiamine does not cross into the brain. Allithiamine which naturally occurs in garlic, and its synthetic counterpart TTFD (thiamine tetrahydrofurfuryl), has been widely used by Dr Lonsdale in his treatment of patients. However, as none of these derivatives have been tested yet in any research studying their effect on Parkinson's or appeared in available anecdotal accounts of success, it is not possible to advise on their use in Parkinson's at this time.

Intramuscular injections

In the research discussed in the previous chapter, thiamine was administered by intramuscular injection. Two advantages of taking B1 by injection are that improvements in symptoms seem to appear quickly, and it is a safer way of taking thiamine for people with problems swallowing.

For many patients, however, their health professionals are not able to give injections on a regular basis and few individuals are trained to administer injections themselves. Dr Costantini also pointed out a contra-indication for patients who are treated with anticoagulants (e.g. Coumadin, Sintrom), and suggested that they did *not* use thiamine injections as they might cause a hematoma.

Oral thiamine HCL

As an alternative to injections, Dr Costantini recommended using oral thiamine. He stressed that this should be B1 hydrochloride (HCL) not B1 mononitrate. Both are synthetic vitamins, but hydrochloride is more water soluble and therefore is not likely to build up in the body. Although low levels of thiamine mononitrate are unlikely to cause any severe problems, the nitrate groups, which are present in thiamine mononitrate molecules, may accumulate in the kidneys and induce kidney stones by forming insoluble nitrate compounds when thiamine is taken in high doses.

The advantage of using oral thiamine HCL is that it is easily available, with a large selection of products to choose from, in either tablets, capsules or powder. Most people use tablets or capsules which are 500 mg each. Make sure it is the 'HCL' version and that it does not contain any other supplements. Some B1 tablets/capsules also contain magnesium and these should be avoided to prevent magnesium overdosing.

Oral versions of thiamine do, however, have drawbacks. The tablet/capsule has quite a journey through the body before it is absorbed. It is swallowed, then digested and absorbed through the lining of the gastrointestinal system where it passes into the smallest blood vessels of the circulatory system and spreads throughout the body. To work correctly, therefore, the thiamine must be able to withstand the highly acidic environment within the stomach, pass through the cells lining the intestines and resist filtration or elimination by the liver before reaching the rest of the body. (https://compoundingrxusa.com/blog/compounding-sublingual-medications/)

Because of this, the oral version of B1 must be taken in rather high doses and several tablets or capsules may be needed to achieve the desired daily dose. As some people have found that taking B1 in late afternoon or evening can interfere with their sleep, the dosage should either be split, taking half the dose with/without breakfast and the rest with/without lunch, or alternatively the complete dose can be taken in the morning.

Dr Costantini advised that the oral version should not be taken with juices but with water only. Some nutritionists also recommend that coffee and tea should be avoided because they contain tannins which can react with thiamine, converting it to a form that is difficult for the body to absorb. Others think the interaction between coffee and tea and thiamine may not be important unless the diet is low in vitamin C. Vitamin C seems to prevent the interaction between thiamine and the tannins in coffee and tea (medlineplus.gov). However, the issues with tea and coffee are probably not relevant, in view of the large doses of thiamine being taken. If there is concern, the B1 could be taken an hour before or after tea/coffee.

Sublingual tablets

One form of thiamine which does not involve the administration of injections or taking high numbers of tablets or capsules is the B1 sublingual tablet. This was not available in Italy when Dr Costantini was advising his patients and consequently was not mentioned by him.

The B1 sublingual tablet is taken by placing it under the tongue where it dissolves rapidly on the mucous membranes beneath the tongue and enters directly into the tiny blood vessels beneath. Sublingual tablets consequently have a more predictable potency. Where oral medications often decrease in potency after being exposed to stomach acids and liver filtrations, sublingual tablets, when taken correctly, dispense the full amount of medication directly into the bloodstream and as a result considerably smaller doses are needed.

Sublingual tablets are also a better format for those who have problems swallowing and/or have digestive issues. The tablet has a rather bitter taste, but most patients find this becomes less noticeable after a few days use.

It is very important that the sublingual tablet is taken correctly, however, and the following procedure is recommended.

1. Drink a glass of water first thing in the morning, (before cleaning your teeth, drinking, or eating anything). This ensures that there is adequate saliva to dissolve the tablet.
2. Wait ten minutes
3. Carefully place the tablet under the tongue. It will dissolve very quickly. Try not to swallow it.
4. Do not eat, drink or clean your teeth for at least 30 to 45 minutes. Food or liquid can wash away a portion of the dose. Do not smoke or chew tobacco for two hours before or after taking the tablet. Both can prevent the mucous membranes in the mouth from properly absorbing the medication.

There are several tablets on the market which purport to be sublingual tablets merely because they dissolve. To the best of my knowledge, the only sublingual B1 tablet currently available is made by 'Superior Source'. This tablet is compounded from thiamine mononitrate, and although we have explained that this is not recommended for oral administration, it should be quite safe when taken sublingually as it does not pass through the digestion and is taken in much smaller doses than oral thiamine.

Websites which sell thiamine in its various forms can be found in 'Useful addresses' at the back of the book.

What is the right dose?

Unfortunately, there is no quick or simple answer to this question, as the dose needed is very person specific. It can be affected by weight, duration of the disease, severity of symptoms and factors so far not known. We do know, however, that if not enough B1 is taken, there will be no improvements and if too much is taken, there will be a temporary worsening of symptoms, though this is quickly rectified by stopping B1 for 1-2 weeks and restarting at a lower dose. Until research clarifies the components that guide individual dosing, the problem must be solved by trial and error. However, my aim here is to present some suggestions and guidance that will hopefully make finding the correct dose easier.

Which dosage?

The dosages which produce improvements in the injection and sublingual forms of thiamine do not appear to vary anywhere near as extensively as thiamine does in its oral form. Those I have suggested below for injection and sublingual are the final doses people have found successful, whereas the start dose I have suggested for the oral version is just that, a dose to start with while monitoring symptoms.

Dr Costantini initially recommended that a therapeutic dose for oral HCL was between 2,000 mg and 4,000 mg. While working with patients around the world via email, however, it came to his attention that patients of Anglo-Saxon origins (Northern Europe and the USA) and Africans required smaller doses to reach the same clinical results compared to his Italian patients. The average range of successful dosages used by people on the Parkinson's forum (https://healthunlocked.com/cure-parkinsons) appears to be between 1,500 mg and 2,500 mg, but in any case it is preferable to start low to check there is no allergic reaction to thiamine and to see whether a low dose might be better for you. In fact, two of the people who have shared their experiences in Chapter 4, found that the oral dose which produced positive results for them was a dose below 200 mg.

Suggested start doses for each of the forms of thiamine -

2 x 50 mg (or 2 x 100 mg) **injectable** solution *per week*

500 mg **oral** thiamine HCL daily (or possibly twice daily, one in the morning and one at lunch time)

1 x 100 mg of **sublingual** B1 on Monday, Wednesday and Friday each week

These are not in any way equivalent doses. It is impossible to suggest comparative potency when the oral version depends so much on a person's gastrointestinal function and their ability to absorb nutrients. These are, therefore, only suggestions for where to start your trial. For some people, even these low doses could be too high, so be alert to the possibility of overdosing symptoms. These will be discussed later. The range for successful oral doses is very broad (100 mg - 4,000 mg) but satisfactory injection doses seem to be either 2 x 50 mg or 2 x 100 mg per week. Few sublingual success doses have been collected so far, but 1 x 100 mg tablet per day is one which has been initially successful for quite a number of people including myself. It is unlikely that more than one tablet will be needed. Over time I have needed to reduce my dosage to avoid overdose symptoms and now take just 3 x 100 mg sublingual tablets *per week*.

Monitor symptoms

How will you know when you have reached the correct dose? Quite simply when symptoms improve. It is very easy, however, to miss these changes, as I know from personal experience. Therefore, to ensure that you do not miss signs of improvement, I suggest you consider using one or more of the following monitoring methods below.

Dr Costantini liked to test his patients' reactions to something called 'the pull test'. Instructions for performing this are as follows-

1. The subject stands comfortably with feet shoulder-width apart and eyes open.
2. The examiner stands behind the subject.
3. The subject is instructed to do whatever it takes to not fall and is told that the examiner will catch them if they do fall.
4. The examiner gives a sudden, brief backward pull to the shoulders of the subject with sufficient force to cause the subject to need to regain his/her balance. The subject is not told when this pull is going to happen.

The steps needed to regain balance are then counted. In a normal response to the pull test, the person either stays steady or takes one or two steps back to avoid falling. A Parkinson's patient, however, will often need to take more before recovering or might need to be assisted to prevent a fall.

Dr Costantini would use the normalising of the pull test as an indication that the correct dose had been found. It can take up to a month on the right dose before the pull test is normalised. In Dr Costantini's opinion, Parkinson's medications did not improve this test, only B1.

You will find short videos on YouTube showing Dr Costantini conducting pull tests with some of his patients under the following titles:

MARCO P PD TWO years after TH
https://youtu.be/yyts9USMTos

Patient 18 PD6 pull test https://youtu.be/YEejV3NmY98

PZ1 Febbraio https://youtu.be/IPxxkCZJbyo

It is a good idea to make 'before' and 'after' videos showing yourself speaking, walking, and performing the pull test. Improvements can be so gradual that even people you live with might not notice the subtle changes. Videos offer the opportunity to watch and compare over a longer period when the extent of the differences can often surprise you.

Another way of monitoring for improvement is to fill in the questionnaire referred to as 'the Unified Parkinson's Disease Rating Scale' (UPDRS). This can be found at https://www.

mdapp.co/unified-parkinson-s-disease-rating-scale-updrs-calcu
lator-523/

This scale is a rating tool used to gauge Parkinson's symptoms in patients. Completing this each week would be one very thorough way of monitoring for changes.

Simply keeping a diary and selecting symptoms to rate would also help. Alternatively, you might ask your friends and/or family, or anyone who sees you frequently and knows you well, to let you know if they think you are looking better. Do not expect to immediately recognise changes yourself. The changes are so gradual and initially so subtle that it is easy to miss them. This could mean that you assume the dose has done nothing for you and move on to a higher level too soon.

Identifying overdose symptoms

One sign that your B1 dose is too high for you could be a worsening of symptoms. Perhaps your constipation, which improved initially, has returned, or a shoulder has become painful once more, or your tremor seems worse, or perhaps a new symptom has emerged. Often people describe feeling jittery or have unexplained anxiety. One person said it was like having had too much coffee. I was watching my young grandson playing with a wind-up toy the other day. If he only turned the winder a little, the toy travelled along briefly and stopped. If he turned and turned the winder until he could not turn it anymore, the toy buzzed around crazily, unable to stop till all the energy was spent. In many ways, that could describe my underdose and overdose signals!

If you suspect the B1 dose is too high for you, immediately stop it for 1-2 weeks or until the symptoms subside, then restart B1 after the short break at a lower dose.

Be patient

It is important to allow an adequate amount of time at each dosage level for improvements to appear. Some people talk of at least six weeks before they noted any changes. You will need to stay at each dosage level for at least two full weeks, and I would recommend four to six weeks to ensure improvements have time to appear and be noted. If you are a lightweight and/or recently diagnosed, you are likely to settle on a lowish dose. Alternatively, if your weight is heavier and/or your symptoms reasonably advanced, you may need a higher dose. A glance through the personal accounts in Chapter 4 will show quite a variation in the dosage that people found successful, particularly when using oral thiamine HCL.

Do not muddy the water

It is often tempting to try various promising therapies at the same time. You are understandably impatient to improve, and you feel that it does not matter which makes you better as long as something does. However, because B1 will only be of benefit if you find the correct dose, you need to be clear what, if anything, is affecting your symptoms. Therefore, when you test

B1, do not increase your medication, add other supplements, or change your regime in any other way until you have established the correct B1 dose for you.

Maintenance

When you have found the dose which for you has produced some symptom improvements, stay on it, and wait patiently. It can take between three and six months for the peak of improvement to manifest.

Taking a break from B1

There are two issues to discuss relevant to using the correct dose long term. One relates to taking breaks from B1 for a short period of time. In the case of intramuscular injections in particular, Dr Costantini found that it could be a good idea, once his patient was stabilized, to take a week's break every two-three months. If the dose has been a little too high, this allows any overdosing to clear. Whichever form of thiamine is taken, if any of the overdose symptoms, described earlier, appear, then it is a good idea to stop the B1 until the symptoms pass.

How long should the break last? Although most of the symptom improvements gained through taking B1 last during a break of several months, many people find that fatigue returns after a very short break. So as a general guide, I would suggest stopping B1 when symptoms worsen or anxiety or jitteriness is felt and restarting B1 again as soon as fatigue reappears. Most long-term users of B1 get to know their own signs of over or under dosing.

Adjusting dosage over time

In the maintenance period when you have found the correct dose, it is quite possible to return to this dosage after the break with no reappearance of overdosing symptoms for a further long period. If the overdose symptoms happen again in a short time, however, it may be necessary to readjust your initial 'correct dose'. Although Dr Costantini suggested that once the right dose had been found, it should not be changed and should always be effective, in several of the personal stories in the next chapter, people talk about needing to adjust their original dosage to maintain the previous benefits.

Taking levodopa medication and other vitamin supplements when taking B1

Thiamine can be safely taken with other supplements and drugs. The patient's regular Parkinson's medication should be continued and indeed, Dr Costantini found that thiamine improved the efficacy of traditional PD medicines. According to Dr Costantini the HDT therapy is not a cure for Parkinson's, but as it is understood currently, it is a co-adjuvant therapeutic measure to use with levodopa therapy, if already prescribed, and that the dosage of the Parkinson's medications should not be altered unless your specialist suggests that you do so.

Dr Costantini also recommended adding other group B vitamins, including folic acid, though he suggested that these should not be added before the correct dosage of B1 was found. This is because multivitamin compounds can contain vitamin B6, and B6 is a facilitator of the peripheral decarboxylase. In people with Parkinson's this may interfere with the amount of levodopa that reaches the brain thereby worsening symptoms. Usually, the levodopa compounds contain inhibitors of such action. However, since this interference may occur even in the presence of inhibitors, it would not be possible to decide whether the best B1 dose had been achieved.

When the correct dose has been found, Dr Costantini also recommended adding a small dose of magnesium. Magnesium is necessary for the activation of thiamine inside the cells and is a co-factor for the activity of various enzymes. Dr Costantini suggested that an extended-release magnesium tablet (375 mg) should be taken just twice a week (www.highdosethiamine.org).

A better alternative to waiting till the right dose is found, is to begin the B-complex and magnesium 2-4 weeks before beginning B1. In this way their addition would not affect finding the best B1 dose.

Safety of high doses of thiamine

High doses of thiamine are safe (Costantini et al 2015), and the literature does not mention adverse thiamine-related effects even at high doses or over very long periods of administration. (Smithline et al 2012 and Meador et al 1993).

Non-responders

Currently, a full understanding of the interactions between thiamine and Parkinson's that result in symptom improvement, does not exist. Until funding can be procured for a rigorous in-depth study, we are limited to theories and hypotheses. Perhaps when it is possible to understand why some people with Parkinson's have such a good reaction to High Dose Thiamine, it will be possible to understand why for others it does not seem to work as well. A crucial goal of the double-blind trial, planned by the Italian research team, is to study the cohort after the trial to understand whether a biomarker exists and to reconstruct the metabolic pathway that leads to specific results.

Dr Costantini said he did not have any patients who did not respond to treatment with thiamine. However, in the Parkinson's forum (www.healthunlocked.com) and the Facebook group "Parkinson's B1 therapy" (https://www.facebook.com/groups/parkinsonsb1therapy/?ref=share), there are people who have not found success with thiamine. I would like to point out some suggestions as to why, for some people, the B1 therapy might not have resulted in symptom improvement so far.

Slowly wins the race

One common error people make, in their keenness to achieve improvements, is to move through the dosage levels too quickly without allowing time for symptom improvements to show at any dosage level. Although positive effects can appear quite quickly when using the injection method, it can take several months with the oral and sublingual form of administration. I would recommend staying at each dose for six weeks to thoroughly test a level before increasing to the next dosage.

Unable to recognise that things are changing

Improvements can also be missed because some people are not prepared for the subtlety of early symptom changes and move to a higher dose, thinking there has been no improvements. Frequently, people do not notice the changes themselves, as I did not at first. Often it is a spouse or friends who point out the changes.

Dr Costantini was disappointed when his patients remarked that there had been little change when he could see great changes. He made short videos of each patient's tremor, walking and the pull test at each visit so that at their next visit he could show them previous videos to compare. One patient said that when he reviewed his videos after a year, he could not believe his eyes and had not realised that so much had improved.

Faulty administration

One problem which happens frequently with the sublingual form of B1 is that the tablets are not taken correctly. I have come across people who chewed them and swallowed them, and a few who spat out the dissolved tablet! As explained in the instructions above, the tablet needs to be put under the tongue and given plenty of time to dissolve, pass through the skin and enter the bloodstream. Every effort should be made not to swallow it until it has had a chance to do this, and the dissolved tablet should definitely not be spat out!

When to stop increasing the dose

Some people notice small improvements and think that if they take more thiamine, they will see bigger improvements. If you increase your dose after you have seen recovery of any symptom, you are likely to cause over-dosing leading to worsening symptoms.

Misinterpreting worsening symptoms

When trying to find their correct B1 dosage, people can misinterpret the cause of any worsening symptoms. Firstly, they may think that they need a higher dose of B1. We are used to increasing doses of medication when symptoms worsen. We do it with our Parkinson's medication and we adopt the same principle when we have a headache. However, B1 dosing does not work in that way. More is not necessarily better. The worsening symptoms are possibly a sign of overdosing, so a reduction in dosage or a break is needed. Secondly, people might not connect the worsening symptoms to B1 and, instead, blame natural progression of their Parkinson's and assume that they need to increase their Parkinson's medication. In fact, Dr Costantini believed that once a patient had established the correct dose of thiamine and was stable with a very good Pull Test response and a very good symptom reduction, this person would never need to increase their other PD medications such as levodopa. Therefore, if symptoms worsen, when taking B1, firstly suspect a B1 overdose and stop taking it for 1-2 weeks to see if symptoms improve.

Gastrointestinal dysfunction

In Chapter 2 I have mentioned the research which suggests that gastrointestinal dysfunction is common in Parkinson's patients, and that this can potentially affect the therapeutic intervention (Pfeiffer 2003). Age too, can affect the intestinal absorption of thiamine, (Baum & Iber 1984, Baker et al 1980). It seems possible, therefore, that this may reduce the effectiveness of oral thiamine for some people and these people might find better success with injections or sublingual tablets.

Other nutrients

The nutritionist Elliot Overton, in a private email, suggested to me that some B1 'non-responders' might not be paying enough attention to other nutrients. He thought that in many cases, thiamine could be intolerable, or even ineffective, without supporting other cofactors when mega-dosing with thiamine. Dr Derrick Lonsdale, known for his research into thiamine, also supports this approach. The other nutrients, which Overton names as becoming deficient when taking high doses of thiamine, are magnesium, occasionally potassium, as well as riboflavin and the other B vitamins. Dr Costantini also included other nutrients in his protocol but took a more conservative approach, giving his patients small amounts of the other B vitamins on the days they received their B1 injections. He also recommended low doses of magnesium (375 mg extended-release tablets twice *a week*) to be taken when the right thiamine dose had been established.

In conclusion

I would like to have been able to end this chapter with a four-step 'quick start' for the High Dose Thiamine protocol. However, there is so much that needs to be understood about every step of the protocol that it would not have explained enough and could have led to confusion and misunderstanding. Consequently, you will need to read the chapter, though, as a reminder, the following brief instructions cover what you need to do to get started on the therapy.

- Choose the form of thiamine you want to use and purchase it.
- Collect monitoring equipment - make videos, fill in UPDRS, start a diary.
- Decide which dose you will start at.
- Monitor, monitor, monitor.

4. Purely Anecdotal

While writing this book, I invited Parkinson's patients who had adopted this therapy to write about their experiences, and this chapter presents the accounts from some of those who replied. They are not, of course, a proportional representation of all who take B1 either in form of thiamine used, experiences or dosages. I must also emphasise that through necessity many are working on their own, without the advice and guidance of a health professional, knowledgeable in this therapy. The stories are anecdotal. They do not necessarily represent the ideal way to approach the therapy. I have included them here, however, because as a society we enjoy learning about the experiences of others, and from them we can gain information, reassurance, guidance, ideas, inspiration and much more.

I have numbered the accounts to make them easier to reference. There is no significance in the order in which they appear, other than that was the order in which they were received. They were collected between October 2021 and January 2022. It is amazing to think that Dr Costantini was based in Italy, but, even after his death, his therapy is benefitting people writing here from Australia, Denmark, France, New Zealand, Sweden, Switzerland, The Philippines, UK and USA.

Most of these stories are from people taking oral thiamine hydrochloride. This is not because oral thiamine is in any way more successful than other forms of thiamine but because the oral B1 became the most popular form to use when injections were not an option for many people and B1 HCL was easily available. My story in Chapter 1 is about my experience with sublingual thiamine. Recently, I have been posting on FaceBook and the Parkinson's forum about using the sublingual version of thiamine and, as a result, more people have started to use this form (#22, #25). There is just one story here from a person using injections (#13). There is also an account from a person whose husband had instant overdose symptoms on even low doses of oral HCL but who eventually found success with low doses of oral B1 mononitrate (#27). There is a huge variation in the length of time the authors of the accounts here have been taking B1, with one having taken B1 for six years while others are sharing the excitement of their initial improvements after just a few weeks.

In their accounts, people list a variety of symptoms which have been affected by B1. In Appendix 1 at the back of the book, you can read a fuller list of symptom improvements sent in by B1 users to the Parkinson's forum (https://healthunlocked.-com/cure-parkinsons).

Two things stand out in these accounts, the determination with which people try and fail and try again, in their attempt to find something that will improve their health, and the joy and gratitude which they show when describing their improvements.

#1 Anya from Oregon, USA wrote...

My symptoms began in 2011 with fatigue and left foot discomfort while wearing footwear. Early in 2012, my left leg drag impeded my hiking adventures, followed soon after with painful toe curling and a mild twitch in the toes of the same foot. I was so busy caring for my parents at the time, I pushed past my symptoms until I could no longer function. By the time I was diagnosed in 2015, I was sleeping away most days and needed a cane (or two) to walk.

I stumbled onto Health Unlocked (Parkinson's forum- https://healthunlocked.com/cure-parkinsons) in 2017 and decided to try High Dose Thiamine therapy. I found improvement within the first month. My energy began to return, toe curling was reduced, and I was able to walk easily without a cane. Some months later the leg drag disappeared (it reappears when I'm very tired). Although I still have tremors, my life is vastly improved because of B1. I have been using it for nearly four years.

My starting dose was 500 mg daily. Every 10 days I increased by 500 mg until settling at 3.5 grams. I remained well on that dosage for about 18 months, then symptoms worsened. I then reduced the B-1 to 1000 mg daily and added magnesium to prevent muscle cramping. Although my need for levodopa has not decreased, it has not increased in 3 1/2 years.

I live an active, independent life. I feel sure that without B-1 I'd have been in a wheelchair by now.

#2 Kia from UK wrote...

I have been taking B1 (3g daily in a divided dose) for almost 4 years and 4 months without any side effects. Almost all my non motor symptoms disappeared within the first few months of starting B1. I am rigidity dominant, and B1 could not resolve my dystonia completely. I had to start a micro dosing with Sinemet and some dystonia recovery training to get rid of my dystonia.

#3 Rob from Florida USA wrote...

I do still use B1. It isn't exactly a night and day difference. I think the benefit I am getting is more in the slowdown of progression and prevention of any levodopa side effects, although my progression has always been slow and never had side effects anyway. I guess you could say I take it more for preventative maintenance. Just for the record, I take 2000 mg per day, though this had varied from 1000 mg to 4000 mg while I was working with Dr Costantini to find the optimal dose. I take a month off every few months, as directed by the good doctor.

#4 Jay from the USA wrote...

I have been taking High Dose Thiamine since March 2018 without interruption. Within the first week or two I noticed my intestinal peristalsis returned to normal after having been sluggish and constipated for some time. Between the third and fourth month I experienced a noticeable improvement in my tremor and motor impairment. These improvements remain in place to the current day.

After starting on some higher doses, I settled on taking 500 milligrams twice daily. Some time ago I reduced that dosage to 500 milligrams once daily.

#5 Roger from UK wrote...

Having been to the neurologist with freezing episodes, tremors and significant leg jerks when resting (I had previously been diagnosed with peripheral neuropathy), the neurologist said I did not have Parkinson's but a neurological movement disorder and offered no treatment. As the symptoms were getting worse and I could see that they would be life changing I decided to investigate myself. I came across Dr Costantini and his followers, via health unlocked, who recommended high dose vit B1. I was highly sceptical but having established that it was unlikely to be dangerous to take a high dose I thought I would give it a go. I bought Solgar vit B1 from Amazon and started taking 4g (4000 mg) per day. Prior to taking B1, my symptoms were occurring every day, but within 2 weeks the freezing episodes stopped, and tremors and jerks reduced significantly to be only a mild prob-lem. I still did not believe taking a vitamin could have such a significant effect so I stopped taking the vitamin. After a few days the symptoms gradually returned and so I took the high dose daily for 14 months. During this period I had only very mild tremors and jerks. However, the symptoms started to get worse after 14 months so, after referring to the Costantini group, I reduced the dose gradually to the point where I now take virtu-ally no vitamin although my symptoms are appearing again. I am not sure where I go from here but I have achieved 2 years free of symptoms and as far as I am concerned this has been a miracle cure. I cannot believe this works for everyone but it has got to be worth giving it a try.

#6 Carol from Nebraska, US wrote...

I started B1 in January 2019. I corresponded with Dr Costantini before he became ill. He started me on 1000 mg. I had severe anxiety and jitteriness. He said to move to 500 mg. Same reac-tion. He then became ill and could no longer respond. I went down to 100 mg and have been at that dose since then. I did try 200 mg several times but always went back to 100 mg. My sense of smell returned, my balance improved, and my handwriting returned to normal.

#7 John of USA wrote...

I started HDT in March 2018 after being diagnosed a year earlier. I did not believe in it but in desperation I gave it a try. It solved all my non-motor issues. I felt improvement after one month but after three months they were very consistent. I started with 2 g a day, 1 g at 8 am and 1 g at 2 pm. One time I tried 4 g but my blood pressure went crazy. (I had never had blood pressure issues before).

Right now I'm at 1g a day for about 2 years, taken after lunch. I use Solgar tablets and I chew them with chocolate. I tried also Vitacost capsules but I do not like to swallow them.

I'm still working due to HDT. I had been at the point of giving up in 2018.

#8 Lyn from UK wrote...

My mum has been on B1 for 10 weeks and yesterday, what a difference! She got up off the couch in the middle part, first go. She seemed full of energy and said that, the day before that, she had felt really well and was walking a lot easier. She is on 2x 500 mg a day.

#9 Deb from New Hampshire/USA wrote...

My name is Deb and I am a person with Parkinson's Disease, diagnosed in 2015 at the age of 57. My symptoms began as hammertoes that caused so much damage that I needed several surgeries before finally getting screws inserted into 3 toes. The PD progressed quickly and within a few years I could not walk or stand without support, could not drive, could barely dress myself and just taking a shower would exhaust me. All types of PD medications caused bad side effects, including Sinemet. At my last appointment with a Movement Disorder Specialist in December 2018, I was told my only option was DBS (Deep Brain Stimulation) brain surgery and was scheduled to begin the approval process.

In a panic, I intensified my online searching for other options, and I stumbled onto a FaceBook group (Parkinson's Disease Fighters United) that was discussing High Dose Thiamine treatment and the members were reporting major reductions in their PD symptoms. And the therapy was inexpensive, low risk and didn't require a doctor's appointment! This was a no-brainer so I quickly placed an online order for thiamine(B1).

I started right away at 2000 mgs/day and within 3 days my balance started improving. Within a week I no longer needed the walker. I had more energy and grew more confident in my abilities each day. Within 3 weeks I was driving again and back at yoga classes. I got my life back! I am not 'cured' of Parkinson's Disease but my quality of life has improved immensely. This therapy may not be a cure but it makes living with the disease a whole lot easier. And choosing vitamins over brain surgery was one of the best decisions I ever made.

I started taking B1 in early 2019. I have tried different doses as high as 3000 mgs/day (made me too jittery) and for about 6 months only took 1000 mgs/day. More recently I am back at 2000 mgs/day which seems to be best for me.

I took a 30-day break after 18 months just to see how I would function without B1. I was ok for about 3 weeks then PD symptoms started returning - stutter steps, unsteady balance and slight tremor. At 4 weeks my PD symptoms were getting worse so I went back on 2000/day and was fine again within a couple of days.

#10 Maria from The Phillipines wrote...

I take 2 grams of B1 per day. It has been a real life changer. I have no more pain, balance issues, constipation, brain fog or masked face. I have improved handwriting, I can now roll over in bed, brush my teeth and a few other symptoms have gone or improved. The best thing is that I can now function even during my 'off' time.

#11 Barbara from USA wrote...

I was diagnosed in June 2021. Although in retrospect I think I've been suffering for about 12 years. Twelve years ago, I had both of my knees replaced. Then this year I had revision surgery on both of my knees. Also, I had a fall that required me to have a quadricep repair this year. I think I was blaming all the stiffness that I had on my knee problems that in fact were probably due to Parkinson's. I also had problems losing my voice and having a very scratchy voice. I lost my sense of smell about 12 years ago as well.

I started on the thiamine regimen about three weeks ago and immediately felt a positive result. I have suffered from depression my whole adult life and have been treated with antidepressants, but I could see that I immediately felt lighter and less apathetic by the next morning. The stiffness was much reduced, and I sometimes forget that I have Parkinson's.

I started by taking 500 mg and increased it by 500 mg every other day until I got to 3,500 mg. At that point I felt the pain and increased stiffness, so I backed off to 3,000 mg a day. I think that is faster than most people seem to increase their dosage but for now that dose seems to work for me.

#12 Carla from USA wrote...

I am a retired Critical Care RN. Probably the most sceptical person ever of such "serendipitous" therapy. But, for me B1 has been a blessing. I was actually diagnosed in 2016, but was symptomatic for a good five years prior at least. As a typical nurse I was ignoring the symptoms, not wanting to believe it was Parkinson's, which I knew in my heart it probably was. My mobility has greatly improved and activities like brushing my teeth, showering, cooking, driving etc have improved. I can use both arms and hands to wash my hair which is huge. Prior to the start of High Dose Thiamine my right arm and hand were nearly non-functional. I am left side dominant. I am no longer dragging my right *foot as I was. I have more energy. I am not 100%, but I am defi-nitely much, much better, and I will take that any day with a huge smile on my face. I can spend the day with my grand-daughter reading and playing games, without saying "grandma's shaky" or "grandma can't do this, that or the other because of Parkinson's". I am thrilled beyond measure with my personal results. And I am forever grateful and thankful for these wonderful results, and to this kind physician who has shared all of this.*

#13 Giorgio from Italy wrote...

In 2009 I had my first episode of tremor in my left arm following bad news, but minor episodes had occurred before. Over the years it continued to worsen. Then in 2013/2014 the tremor in my arm was continuous, I was always tired, I struggled to work, I had neck pain, a little sciatica, stiff muscles and rigid facial expressions. However, due to non-motor symptoms such as constipation, often vomiting, dizziness, and burning of the oesophagus, due to a hiatal hernia, I had not attributed it to Parkinson's. So I did not go to a neurologist until 2014.

My first neurologist gave me three examinations, brain MRI, blood tests and Dat-scans. My Dat-scan was not like that of a healthy person. At this point I came across the videos of Doctor Costantini on the Web and read of his use of high doses of thiamine hcl, I took them to my family doctor who is a smart guy. He watched the videos and quickly realized what they meant. He said "In your shoes, with Parkinson's disease, I would try some-thing like this right away to see if it works and does what it promises, as it doesn't have any major side effects, but then go to this neurologist and follow what he says". He handed me 6 injections of 100 mg of thiamine hcl and told me to administer one twice a week with the precaution of being careful of hives or allergic reactions. I had already taken oral thiamine hcl for a few days before I had seen the doctor, but after the first injection the muscle stiffness started to melt and more so after the second. After the injections, the most noticeable gains are in the first few weeks, because then your energy returns, you move more, you are more cheerful and a spiral is triggered where a physical improvement leads to an improvement in mood.

Following the advice of my family doctor, I phoned Costantini's number. Much to my surprise he answered me in person and told me to make an appointment at his office, which I did promptly and after about a month I had a consultation with him where I took a full UPDRS test and he made a short video which served to document progress over time.

That was September 2015 and since then for six years I have had two or three 100 mg intramuscular injections of thiamine HCL almost every week with no side effects other than occasionally having a little difficulty and restlessness in the evening, which is quickly resolved by missing a few injections. The fixed dose makes no sense with B1. Sometimes I take a week's break, sometimes I feel the need to take three a week. It is something that you learn by using it. I regulate myself on these three symptoms: tiredness, agitation, little sleep. The base dose remains 100 mg twice per week.

Dr. Costantini added levodopa to my therapy with the thiamine hcl, explaining that levodopa is complementary and necessary to help the reduced dopamine production in the remaining brain cells that survived the disease. Surviving brain cells are partly healthy, partly dying, and some nearing death on a gradual basis. Thiamine helps these last two categories on an energetic level, and this explains the improvements, but it is not a cure. This is just a simplification of what he said and to explain this to me further he made some sketches.

Six years on I am a little stiffer at night and I have added a few points to my UPDRS score but as soon as I stop the thiamine, I immediately feel the difference in muscle strength and the levodopa is less functional and I cannot do without the B1.

I saw Dr. Antonio Costantini 4 times in 2 and a half years. He was an excellent professional and knew the sick very well, so much so that he immediately understood your condition. He treated you as a person to help, not a body to be treated. Dr Costantini was very positive and having found this therapy he wanted to use it and make it known as much as possible. When a patient came back and got better, like me, he was very happy. I think his basic motivation was a sense of duty and help. I always came out of every visit with him with great hope and enthusiasm, sure that I would not get worse and so it has been, well almost. A heartfelt thanks to Dr. Antonio Costantini and his staff.

#14 Larry from USA wrote...

I found Dr. Costantini to be a caring and wonderful mentor in my B1 experience. He always emailed me back within 4-6 hours from Italy. It took about 4-5 weeks for the B1 therapy to take hold. When it did my children asked me "how I cured my Parkinson's?" That was 4-5 years ago I think. I have not been able to get my B1 supply recently and my right hand tremor has reoccurred. When the supply chain over at Vita Cost is fixed, I should regain my former status. I can only tolerate capsules.

#15 Robert from France wrote...

My PD feels a bit weird. It is like all the symptoms came at once after several operations on my bladder. The doctors deny that there is any link but I have my doubts. Anyway, I got pretty much all the symptoms you can think of - posture, aching muscles, shuffling, stone face, isolation in my little world, shaking hands, difficult to talk, etc

I discovered B1 and have taken 3Grams per day for the last two years. What a change! I obviously know I have Parkinson's, but the improvement is enormous.

My French neurologist does not believe it can make a difference even if my tests show no degradation whatsoever in the last two years.

I went to Italy to meet one of the members of the team who devised this B1 protocol, and I plan to go there once a year.

My speech is not perfect (depending on the moment) but if the situation remains stable, I am fine.

#16 Alayne from France wrote...

I was diagnosed with PD (Parkinson's Disease) aged 54 on Nov 30th 2015, without any warning, I had no symptoms to speak of. I had an under-active thyroid so had put on weight, got a bit stiff and slowed up. (Classic PD it seems as well). I worked in Care and had clients with PD so I had some idea of it, but my clients were all in their late 70's and older and so sometimes it was hard to tell if they were slow due to PD or age.

I decided to change my life and its hectic pace. Obviously my job had to go as I was sicker than a lot of my clients who were just old and in need of assistance with daily tasks. By Sept 2016 I had moved from London where I lived with my 3 sons and bought a house in rural France with a holiday home for my income, leaving my sons behind and living alone for the first time in my life! The change in pace was to suit me. In the 6 months before I arrived, I had lost some 28lbs in weight and had resumed running again. The rural life is very physical, I have two dogs. I walk twice a day-rain or shine, I have a large garden that needs tending, I grow my own fruit and veg, I chop logs in winter for my log burners. In summer months I have a swimming pool that needs cleaning etc and I also swim.

I was prescribed PD meds within 5 minutes of my diagnosis but I decided to wait until I needed them. I started on Azilect by April 2016 as I was told it was believed it protected the brain. By May 2018 I had read of Dr Costantini's work with Thiamine and saw some of his video's. These made me cry. To see the improvements patients had achieved was quite remarkable.

I made videos of myself walking and talking as a part of my research into B1 to see if it could help. I noted my aches/pains/difficulties in minute detail so I could refer back when needed and I regularly updated my diary entries - which have proved good for this - so I could judge my improvements. I emailed with Dr Costantini and he helped me with my doses etc. I started on 500 mg twice a day with the intention of getting to 1500 mg twice a day- this was the dose the Dr had other patients on.

I had improvements nearly immediately which was fab. I even had Dr Costantini tell me I had lost my poker face when I sent him new videos. And I had, I looked younger which was a huge boost to my morale. But it was up and down. I couldn't get my dose right. I would stop for a few days or week to 'detox'. On a re-start I could feel my body relax and unlock, which is just amazing after being so rigid all the time, then slowly I would lock up again and my knees would go 'bendy' and not lock. I would also get incredible sweats and a 'running out of fuel' feeling.

I decided to detox for longer and come back at a much lower dose and increase slower, I realised my dose was going to be a lot less than 500 mg once a day. It took me over a year but I knew from the bad reactions that I was responding so it was just a case of dose adjustment.

I have now been on my dose for over two years – I take 1000 mg a week spread over 5 days so that's 200 mg Monday to Friday with Saturdays & Sundays off. I have found the days off just as important otherwise I end up having to detox again. I have a 'fluttery' feeling inside if I overdose and my trigger finger returns if I need B1. It is very fine tuning indeed.

I would say I am in better shape now than I have been for many years and that includes before diagnosis. With the weight gain I was unable to run and flexibility was hampered. Now I take yoga classes and am able to relax my body through yoga and conscious breathing, I run 2-3 times a week, I have learnt to swim again. When I arrived here my right arm had become so weak I could not get it over my head for front crawl. I have not fallen for best part of two years (I can't remember my last fall). I can write again, not pretty but a lot better. My right arm works and joins in with tasks (which is great because my left arm is uncoordinated). I can dance around my kitchen too. I feel stronger in my body.

I am slow, but that may also be because I am careful. I find if I try to multi-task it can go wrong so I tend to be precise and hence slow. I use a stick when shopping but that is mostly because people cut me up and my balance can be off if I stop too quickly, and the stick enables me to push off without hesitation. I added slow release madopor to my regime in June 2019 as per Dr Costantini's instructions and have remained on 2 tablets per day-my neuro wanted me to take 3 a day and I tried but it was too many and interfered with my sleep and brought back the sweats, nausea and exhaustion. I was able to cut out the third tablet with no issue. My prescription has been the same for two and half years now, Dr Constantini believed B1 helps to keep medication low and stop dyskinesia and I pray that it does.

#17 Peggy from Arizona wrote...

I have had PD for three years. I initially started with Levodopa but did not like how it made me feel, so I stopped taking it. I decided to do some research on alternative remedies and came across Dr. Costantini's webpage. I liked what I read and decided to try B1 therapy. I started with one 500 mg capsule per day and worked up to two 500 mg capsules per day – one in the morning and one in the afternoon. The biggest benefit I experience is the elimination of debilitating fatigue. Recently, due to the progression of my fatigue symptoms, I increased my dosage to 2000 mg per day – two capsules in the morning and two capsules in the afternoon – and my fatigue is again gone. The brand I take is Vitacost B1 HCI 500 mg capsule.

#18 Roy from USA wrote...

I was diagnosed in 2012. Four years ago, I started taking 4g of B1 daily. The positive improvements since then - I have no bradykinesia (slowness of movement), I can cut my food with a knife, I have no button difficulties, I can brush my teeth now without needing an electric toothbrush, I have more strength. Getting in and out of bed and turning over is easier. I no longer have constipation. Parkinson's progression has stopped and B1 has suppressed most motor and non-motor symptoms. I am now entering my 9th year post diagnosis and have not fallen, not once, since starting B1, to the surprise of my neurologist.

#19 MJ from New Zealand wrote...

I was diagnosed in July 2020 with PD. My symptoms were and still are pretty mild. My main symptoms are visible tremor in my

left leg, freezing of gait, stiffness in fingers on the left hand, tiredness, my left arm doesn't swing, and I have brain fog.

I started taking B1 in December 2020 at 30 mg for a week then I
increased to 500 mg for a month, then 1500 mg for 4 months, 2 g
for a month then 2.5 g because I started getting dystonia in my
left foot and my toes curled. The tremor on my left leg has
become more frequent since diagnosis but not by much so that
could be due to my B1 dose being too high. The brain fog and
energy levels have improved significantly. Dystonia didn't
improve at 2.5 g so I stopped for a week and resumed at 1.5 g and
started taking Magtein. The dystonia then resolved.

I've been on 1.5 g for three months so far. It seems to be a good
dose for me. Improvements I've experienced are in energy levels
and brain fog. I also don't have constant dystonia anymore. My
gait still freezes but not so obvious most of the time.

#20 Fabrice from Canada wrote...

My mother was diagnosed with PD 1.5 years ago. Initial
symptoms were slowness, tremors on left side, numbness in left
leg, depression, memory issues etc. We first tried Mucuna but she
could not digest it (She has severe gastritis related to B12 auto-
immune deficiency). Her symptoms were getting worse in the
first 6 months, and only exercise seemed to be helping. She was
put on Sinemet and the Drs wanted to add Carbidopa. Given my
dad had severe PD (he passed earlier this year), she knew she
wanted to limit/get off the meds if she could, so increasing
Sinemet and taking Carbidopa was not what she wanted to do.

Vitamin B1 HCL was a game changer for her. We started at 250 mg and increased (doubled every 3-4 days more or less) and each time looked at symptoms. Now she is at 1.75-2.25 g a day and we started noticing the effect really around 1.5 g. The B1 gave her her energy back and addressed quite a few of her symptoms.

#21 Padgett from Texas USA wrote...

I was diagnosed when I was 37. I'm 43 now. It took four neurologists to figure out what was wrong with me. They had to do genetic testing because my MRIs kept coming back normal. I take 1 and a 1/2 (Levodopa) 3 times a day.

I started the vitamin B1 at 500 mg for a month and could tell a slight difference with my hand that kept turning. When I upped my dose to a 1000 mg, my hand didn't turn as much, and my foot stopped gripping the floor. My doctor wanted to put me on some more medication, but I just didn't want to do that, so I now take 1500 mg a day and I feel great. My mom has severe tremors so I also started her on the B1 500 mg a day for a month. Then I upped her dose of B1 to 1000 mg and she doesn't shake anymore.

#22 Joyce from Texas USA wrote...

I was diagnosed on 9/13/2021. Symptoms of slow movements, freezing, tremors on left leg, depression, anxiety. I was an emotional reck prior to starting HDT therapy. I tried the B1 orally, but my stomach can't tolerate it. Luckily, I found

Daphne's post about the sublingual form. Currently I am taking 100 mg sublingual form twice a day. It helps me keep anxiety and depression at bay. It gives me energy and strength, it also keeps my brain sharp, and brain fog away.

#23 Wanda from Kentucky USA wrote...

I've been diagnosed for 3½ years and only take B1. I had the tests, push pull, memory check etc about six months ago and did fair. I only have slight tremors on my left side. I have been taking 500 mg B1 for about a year. The B1 is definitely keeping me off prescription meds.

#24 Keri from Wisconsin USA wrote...

My husband, who has Parkinson's, has just started 500 mg of B1 at breakfast. He was diagnosed with PD five years ago. So far so good with the B1. His tremors have been reduced, his voice has gotten stronger, he has more energy, moves more quickly, and has no more constipation.

#25 Ikka from Sweden wrote...

I am a 66-year-old male from Stockholm in Sweden. I was diagnosed eight years ago. My current medication is 600 mg Madopar, 200 mg Mucuna and 1 mg Rasagiline. I hope I can reduce this amount. I don't have a tremor, but I have some dyski-nesia and wonder if this is because of too much levodopa medication.

I've been using b1 thiamine hcl for about two years. My dosage has been between 1 - 2 grams daily. More than that seems to make me feel jittery and uncomfortable. It is hard to say exactly what symptom relief it has given me. Anyway, I've used thiamine for about two years trying to establish the best dosage for me and not being really satisfied of the results. Then I read Daphne's information about the sublingual b1. I bought it and have taken one tablet (100 mg) for three days now. I'm surprised to say this, but I can feel more positive effect already than I had from the oral b1 in two years. And I don't think this is imagina-tion or placebo either. I have much more energy now and I feel much more normal in my body. I feel "all systems go". The coming weeks will be very interesting.

#26 Rick from Denmark wrote...

I was diagnosed in 2012 and take 3 x 100/25 levodopa medication per day. I've been taking B1 thiamine hcl since last Easter, increasing the dosage slowly from 500 mg to my current dosage of 3 g per day. The results have been variable but my neurologist thinks that my movements were greatly improved, though the tremor is more stubborn to effect.

#27 Gail wrote...

Jay was diagnosed 12/29/21 at the age of 69 (less than a month before he turned 70). He weighed about 156 pounds (not a big man).

I must apologize that my notes for the first few months are not very good. This is my first entry: 2-15-2021 Started High Dose B1 Thiamine Therapy 1000 mg at breakfast and 500 mg at lunch. He had GREATLY increased anxiety and left leg/foot tremor.

We gave the B1 a rest for a couple of weeks. We started again at a lower dose. I am sorry this is where things get murky. I know we tried lower doses of the HCL decreasing to 500 mg twice daily and lower. (I just didn't keep very good records.)

Jay would take a B1 break anywhere from 5 days to 2 weeks before restarting at a lower dose.

The month of March we put Jay on the B1 Thiamine Mononitrate and had really good results. However, by April 14, 2021 I took Jay off Thiamine Mononitrate because it wasn't the preferred type of B1 Thiamine and I didn't want to make a mistake.

April 17, 2021 Jay started Now Brand of B1 Thiamine with just 25 mg at breakfast and lunch. We stopped this because even at this low dose his anxiety and tremor were greatly increased.

May 5, 2021 Jay started BariMelts B1 Thiamine, 12.5 mg twice a day.

May 8 we decided to have Jay to take the two pills (total of 25 mg) 5 days a week and one pill (12.5 mg) 2 days a week. That didn't work, too much anxiety and tremor. Most of the rest of the month we were on and off B1 trying to find the correct dosage and frequency which ended up with a schedule of Monday, Wednesday, Friday 12.5 mg; Tuesday/Thursday 25 mg and nothing on the weekends. And continued this throughout the month of June. At some point we also tried the sublingual B1 Thiamine and that was too strong for him.

July 13, 2021 Jay restarted the B1 Thiamine Mononitrate 25 mg twice daily. My notes for July 14 say "we laughed a lot on our walk and at breakfast. He said that he feels really good on our morning walks."

So July was when we finally found the right "type" of B1 and the right dosage for him.

There has been conflicting thoughts regarding the Thiamine Mononitrate. It isn't the exact type of B1 that Dr. Costintini had his patients on but was there really a reason for not using this one? I don't know. I "talked" with knowledgeable people on the healthunlocked forum who helped me work through all of this. I have read that B1 Thiamine Mononitrate is water soluble and other places have said it isn't. I have read that you should not exceed a certain amount. All I know is that this is the form of B1 that is working for Jay and if there is an amount not to exceed then he is under that amount.

Our schedule for taking B1 Thiamine Mononitrate is 25 mg with breakfast and lunch and he skips one day a week completely. Occasionally he will skip another dose if we have a busy/crazy day. The 25 mg amount is approximate since I have to cut each pill into quarters, but it is working!!!

One more thing, I think the reason it took us 5 months to get to the correct dose for Jay was because he was so newly diagnosed and because he is not a very big man.

If anyone wants to give this B1 Thiamine Mononitrate a try, please do your own research and make sure it's a good fit for you.

#28 Jérôme from Switzerland wrote...

After discovering the therapy browsing on the Internet, I decided to give it a try because my Parkinson symptoms were worsening (constipation, difficulties in swallowing, shuffling my feet, fatigue...). So I began in June 2021 ordering thiamine powder (Prescribed for Life) from the USA. I was really keen on using the product because I was not happy with my traditional medication (Requip). Having bought small scales, I could start the therapy. For the first two weeks of my treatment I took 500 mg in the early morning, then two weeks later I took two doses of 500 mg before breakfast and after lunch for one month. I started noticing little changes but nothing extraordinary, that's why I went on with the therapy. Therefore, I upped the dose to 1500 mg in total again for one month and then to 2000 mg per day still in two doses and for 4 weeks. At this stage I did not feel well and did not know what to do. After pondering over it, I stopped for one week and started back at 1000 mg. I had simply halved the previous dose. It was at the end of October when suddenly I felt rejuvenated since I could move normally again without slowness, I could swallow normally again, could move the fingers of my left hand and my balance was much better. I was so happy. Then a few weeks later, I decided to try B1 sublingual because I needed a change; I started in November then went on through December with one tablet of 100 mg per day, but recently I have not been feeling so well being anxious and walking with difficulty. Now, I am taking two B1 sublingual tablets in order to feel better. Is it the solution, I do not know? Maybe you could help me in this matter.

Author's note: I suggested to Jérôme that his worsening symptoms at one tablet per day were probably an overdose sign and that instead off increasing his dose he should try a reduced dose of six or five tablets a week. He should, however, take a break first to clear the B1 overdose in his system.

#29 Anne from USA wrote...

A few months ago, I started taking thiamine hcl supplements. I started at 500 mg a day, and after six weeks went up to 1,000 mg a day, and then after another six weeks I am now taking 1,500 mg a day. Today I had my annual neurology visit and the doctor said that my scores have improved over last year's visit. My fatigue is significantly reduced, and so is my anxiety. I am more talkative and more animated. I am laughing more. My tremor is reduced, muscle tightness reduced and I play the piano with more fluency.

#30 Ashe from UK/Mother from Australia wrote...

I live in the UK and my mother lives in Australia. Due to Covid I haven't yet been able to visit home since October 2019 so all my observations are based on our daily phone calls. My mother was diagnosed early 2021 after a year of a mystery illness that was misdiagnosed as anxiety. Once we had the name 'Parkinson's' then we were able to start looking for answers.

I heard about B1 and looked through the videos of Dr Costantini and started to talk to Mum about what I was learning. Mum thankfully agreed to try taking 250 mg of B1 HCL and over time we have increased to 1000 mg at one stage. We have tried 700 mg and 800 mg and so far are settled on 500 mg. This is where Mum feels she has reduced fatigue, more energy and few internal tremors.

My Mum's symptoms included an intense feeling of wanting to cut her left hand or arm off and heavy fatigue. She would lie down and do relaxation exercises and although they would help it would take 45 minutes to get back to some kind of normality. Now with B1 she hardly ever feels an internal tremor and certainly never wants to remove a limb. This is a massive change. Also, she has no real fatigue anymore and is back to living an active life.

5. In Conclusion

High Dose Thiamine is a therapy of huge benefits. As we have seen from the published research and the many anecdotal reports, it has improved Parkinson's symptoms by as much as 70% for many, and can at least slow, if not halt progression. It also improves symptoms whatever stage of Parkinson's has been reached. It is inexpensive (my tablets cost £8 a year), is easily acquired in a variety of forms and is safe to use.

There is one aspect of the therapy, however, that does present some difficulty. If the dosage is too low, no improvement will be achieved, but alternatively, if the dosage is too high it can cause symptoms to temporarily worsen. In Chapter 3, I have been as clear and as detailed as possible in describing how to adopt the protocol and especially how to recognise overdose signs, but I know from personal experience, that it is difficult to see your own situation objectively enough to always make the right decisions about whether a dose needs to be increased or decreased.

Future research may discover aspects which will help predict appropriate dosing.

At this current time, many people with Parkinson's are trying High Dose Thiamine on their own, as it is difficult if not impossible to find a health professional experienced in the therapy. To have a novel treatment accepted by the medical profession, it is necessary to produce a rigorous, double-blind, placebo-controlled, multi-based study supporting the hypothesis. The Italian team which produced the available research on thiamine and Parkinson's, have planned such a study but have so far been unsuccessful in getting the funding necessary to carry it out. There is a sense of urgency for this funding to be found, and for neurologists, doctors and Parkinson's nurses to acquaint themselves with this therapy. Many people will have received a diagnosis of Parkinson's while you have read this book, and face a disease, which will be with them for the rest of their lives, and for which there is no medication that will treat the cause, or even slow its progression. As an adjunct therapy, High Dose Thiamine offers much which can make life easier for those people. We need the study to be funded so that drug administrations will give the therapy approval and then trusted medical channels could supervise the proper therapy use.

If you feel you would like to support the funding of such a research project please go to gofundme.

Appendices

Symptom improvements when using B1

Members of the Parkinson's forum, 'Cure Parkinson's' on https://healthunlocked.com/cure-parkinsons, who were using the B1 therapy, were asked to list any improvements they had noticed. These are some of the symptom improvements mentioned which are gathered here under headings.

Non-motor symptoms

Mood

Anxiety reduced or eliminated

Depression reduced or eliminated

Hope for the future improved

Frustration much reduced

Mood improved and mood swings reduced

Willingness to socialise returned

Hopelessness reversed

Apathy reduced or eliminated

Cognitive ability

Brain fog/focus/clarity improved up to 100%

Concentration improved

Improved memory

A return of lost creativity

Sense of smell

Ability to taste and smell returned

Sleep

Improved sleep both in length and quality

Bodily functions

Improvement in gut problems

Urinary incontinence and urgency down to as low as zero

Constipation significantly reduced or eliminated

Fatigue

Fatigue reduced, energy levels increased, endurance improved

Ability to do things after work instead of going home and having to go to bed

Quicker recovery from hard workouts and aerobic exercise

Pain
———

Pain in all areas, neck, back, arms, legs, feet etc reduced or eliminated

Motor symptoms

Gait
———

Gait improved, arm swing returned and shuffling reduced

Ability to do without a walker or cane/walking stick

Walking speed increased with stability and ability to go greater distances

Strength in legs improved

Dragging of feet and legs reduced

Going from not being able to walk, to being able to walk.

Stooped posture improved

Postural instability
————————————

Balance and stability much improved

Push test improvements to a quicker balance response

No longer need to grab onto things to maintain balance

Hands
————

Handwriting/typing/mouse usage increased in speed

Using hands to do things not previously possible

Easier to snap fingers once more

Clapping possible again

Hand strength improved

Movement in general

Bradykinesia/slow motion reduced or eliminated

Movements more fluid

Easier turning in bed

Getting in and out of bed is easier

Able to rise from a seated position unassisted and easily

Able to use stairs normally again

Freezing reduced or eliminated

Flexibility improved

Improved co-ordination

Rigidity

Reduced stiffness

Smiling right up to the eyes again

Masked face normalised

Ability to exercise with greater ease

Dystonia reduced or eliminated

Toe curling reduced

Tremor

Tremor of hands, arms, legs, fingers, toes, feet, head, mouth and jaw reduced to as low as zero.

Twitching reduced or eliminated.

Dyskinesia reduced as low as zero

Voice and swallowing

Improved voice volume, projection and clarity

Improved swallowing ability and confidence

Drooling reduced or eliminated

Other

Hallucinations reduced or eliminated

Muscle cramps reduced

General

Significant slowing or halting of disease progression

'On time' increased, 'off time' decreased

Improvement to a state better than when originally diagnosed

Being able to continue working instead of being forced to retire

Reduction in inflammation

A general feeling of well being

Reduced dosage of Parkinson's medication

Feeling as though you now have a future to look forward to rather than declining health and abilities

An ability to sometimes forget that you have Parkinson's

References

Bager P, Hvas C L, Rud C L, Dahleerup J F. (2021) Randomised clinical trial: high-dose oral thiamine versus placebo for chronic fatigue in patients with quiescent inflammatory bowel disease. *Aliment Pharmacol Ther* 2021,53(1);79-86. Doi;10.1111/apt.16166

Baker H, Frank O, Jaslow S P. (1980) Oral versus intramuscular vitamin supplementation for hypovitaminosis in the elderly. *J Am Geriatr Soc* 28 (1); 42-45

Baum R A, Iber F L. (1984) Thiamine - the interaction of aging, alcoholism, and malabsorption in various populations. *World Rev Nutr Diet*, 44;85-116

Brandis K A, Homes I F, England S J, Sharm N, Kukreja L, DebBurman S K. (2006) Alpha-synuclein fission yeast model: concentration-dependent aggregation without plasma membrane localization or toxicity. *J Mol Neurosci* 2006;28;179-191

Costantini A, Pala M I, Compagnoni L, Colangeli M. (2013) Case report: High-dose thiamine as initial treatment for Parkinson's disease. *BMJ Case Reports*. Published online Aug 28 2013. Doi 10.1136/bcr-2013-009289

Costantini A, Pala M I, Colangeli M, Savelli S, (2013 A). Thiamine and spinocerebellar ataxia type 2. *BMJ Case reports*. Doi.org/10.1136/bcr-2012-007302

Costantini A, Giorgi R, D'Agostino S, Pala M I. (2013 B). High Dose Thiamine improves the symptoms of Friedreich's ataxia, *BMJ Case Reports* doi.org/10.1136/bcr-2013-009424

Costantini A, Nappo A, Pala M I, Zapppone A, (2013 C). High Dose Thiamine improves fatigue in multiple sclerosis. *BMJ Case Rep.* 2013:bcr2013009144. Doi: 10/1136-2013-009144

Costantini A, Pala M I. (2013 D). Thiamine and fatigue in inflammatory bowel diseases. An open-label pilot study. *Journal of Alternative and Complementary Medicine*, vol 19 no 8 pp 704-708.

Costantini A, Pala M I, Tundo S, Matteucci P. (2013 E) High Dose Thiamine improves the symptoms of fibromyalgia. *BMJ Case Rep.* doi:10.1136/bcr-2013-009019

Costantini A, Pala M I, Catalano M L, Notarangelo C, Careddu P. (2014 A) High Dose Thiamine improves fatigue after stroke: a report of three cases. *Journal of alternative and complementary medicine* vol 20, no 9, pp 683-685.

Costantini A, Pala M I. (2014 B) Thiamine and Hashimoto's thyroiditis. A report of three cases. *Journal of alternative and complementary medicine* vol 20, no 3, pp 208-211.

Costantini A, Pala M I, Grossi E, Mondonico S, Cardelli L E, Jenner C, Proietti S, Colangeli M, Fancellu R. (2015) Long-term treatment with High Dose Thiamine in Parkinson's Disease: An open-label pilot study. *The Journal of Alternative and Complementary Medicine.* Vol 21. Number 1222, 2015, pp 740-747 Doi. 10.1089/acm.2014.0353

Costantini A, Trevi E, Pala M I, Fancellu R. (2016 A) Thiamine and dystonia 16, *BMJ case reports*, 2016;bcr-2016-216721 doi: 10.1136/bcr-2016-216721

Costantini A, Trevi E, Pala M I, Fancellu R. (2016 B). Can long-term thiamine treatment improve the clinical outcomes of myotonic dystrophy type 1? *Neural Regeneration Research*, vol 11, no 9, pp 1487-1491

Costantini A, Laureti T, Pala M I, Colangeli M, Cavalieri S, Pozzi E, Brusco A, Salvarani S, Serrati C, Fancellu R. (2016 C). Long-term treatment with thiamine as possible medical therapy for Friedreich ataxia. *J Neurol* 263 no11:pp 2170-2178

Costantini A, Tiberi M, Zarletti G, Pala M I, Trevi E. (2018 A) Oral High Dose Thiamine improves the symptoms of chronic cluster headache. *Case reports in Neurological Medicine* Article ID 3901619 doi.org/10.1155/2018/3901619

Costantini A. (2018 B). High Dose Thiamine and essential tremor. *BMJ Case Reports* vol 2018;bcr2017223945. Doi 10.1136/bcr-2017-223945

Goedert M (2001). Alpha-synuclein and neurodegenerative diseases. *Nat Rev Neurosci* 2(7);492-501. Doi.10.1038/35081564

Gold M, Hauser R A, Chen M F. (1998). Plasma thiamine deficiency associated with Alzeimer's disease but not Parkinson's disease. *Metab Brain Dis.* 13;43-53.

Jhala S S, Hazell A S. (2011) Modelling neurodegenerative disease pathophysiology in thiamine deficiency: consequences of impaired oxidative metabolism. *Neurochem Int* 2011;2013,248-260

Jimenez-Jimenez F J, Molina J A, Hermanz A et al. (1999) Cerebrospinal fluid levels of thiamine in patients with Parkinson's disease. *Neuosci Lett* 271;33-36

Kordower J H, Olanow C W, Dodiya H B, Chu Y, Beach T G, Adler C H, Halliday G M, Bartus R T. (2013) Disease duration and the integrity of the nigrostriatal system in Parkinson's disease. *Brain Volume* 136 Issue 8, 2419-2431. //doi.org/10.1093/brain/awt192

Lonsdale D (2006) A review of the biochemistry, metabolism and clinical benefits of thiamine and its derivatives. *eCAM* 2006,3(1)49-59. Doi:10.1093/ecam/nek009

Lonsdale D (2021) www.hormonesmatter.com/high-dose-thiamine-parkinsons-disease/

Lu'o'ng Kv, Nguyen L T. (2012) Thiamine and Parkinson's disease. *J Neurol Sci* 316;1-8

Lu'o'ng Kv, Nguyen L T. (2012) The beneficial role of thiamine in Parkinson Disease: preliminary report. *J Neurol Res* 2:211-214

Lu'o'ng Kv, Nguyen L T. (2013) The beneficial role of thiamine in Parkinson Disease. *CNS Neurosci Ther* 19(7); 461-468. Doi: 10.1111/cns.12078

Meador K, Loring D, Nichols M, Zamrini E, Rivner M, Posas H, Thompson E, Moore E. (1993). Preliminary findings of High Dose Thiamine in dementia of Alzeimer's type. *J Geriatr Psychiatry Neurol.* Oct-Dec;6(4);222-229 doi; 10.1177/089198879300600408.

Merkin-Zaborsky H, Ifergane G, Frisher S, Valdman S, Herishanu Y, Wirguin I. (2001) Thiamine-responsive acute neurological disorders in nonalcoholic patients. *Eur Neurol* 45;34-37.

Mizuno Y, Matuda S, Yoshino H et al (1994). An immunohistochemical study on alpha-ketoglutarate dehydrogenase complex in Parkinson's disease. *Ann Neurol* 35:204-210

Onodera K, (1987). Effects of decarboxylase inhibitors on muricidal suppression by L-dopa in thiamine deficient rats. *Arch Int Pharmacodyn Ther* 285;263-276

Parkinson J. (1817) An essay on the shaking palsy. *J Neuropsychiatry Clin Neuroscience* 2002, 14:223-236. Discussion 2.

Pfeiffer R F. (2003) Gastrointestinal dysfunction in Parkinson's disease. *Lancet Neurol* 2 (2);107-116

Poewe W, Antonini A, Zijlmans J C, Burkhard P R, Vingerhoets F. (2010). Levadopa in the treatment of Parkinson's disease: an old drug is still going strong. *Clin Interv Aging*, Sept 7;5:229-238. //doi:10.2147/cia.s6456.

Sjoquist B, Johnson H A, Neri A, Linden S. (1988) The influence of thiamine deficiency and ethanol on rat brain catecholamines. *Drug Alcohol Depend* 22;167-193.

Smithline H A, Donnino M, Greenblatt D J, (2012) Pharmacokinetics of high dose oral thiamine hydrochloride in healthy subjects. *BMC Clin Pharmacol* 2012;12:4

Abbreviations

HCL - hydrochloride

HDT - High Dose Thiamine

FSS - Fatigue Severity Scale

PD - Parkinson's Disease

UPDRS - Unified Parkinson's Disease Rating Scale

Useful websites and addresses

The official site for Dr Antonio Costantini's research -

https://highdosethiamine.org/

The Unified Parkinson's Disease Rating Scale -

https://www.movementdisorders.org/MDS-Files1/PDFs/
Rating-Scales/MDS-UPDRS_English_FINAL.pdf

https://www.mdapp.co/unified-parkinson-s-disease-rating-
scale-updrs-calculator-523/

Sublingual B1 available from -

https://www.pureformulas.com/no-shot-b-1-100-mg-100-
dissolvable-tablets-by-superior-source

gofundme

https://www.gofundme.com/f/high-dose-thiamine-protocol

Thiamine injections available from -

homoempatia.eu Versandapotheke
Die Kosmos Apotheke Reform Inhaber Sükrü Aydogan e.Kfm.
Reinhard-Mannesmann-Weg 3
39116 Magdeburg
Fax: +493917 2767729
E-Mail:service@homoempatia.eu

Acknowledgments

My first thanks are to my husband, David, who has seen little of me for the past six months and who kindly proof-read the book for me.

I also wish to thank Marco Colangeli and Dr Roberto Fancellu, close colleagues of Dr Costantini, who have supported this project and supplied information when required. They have been kind enough to check that the information I have written and the advice I have given is in keeping with Dr Costantini's practice. My thanks also go to Marco for writing the foreword to the book.

I also extend 'un grand merci' to Jérôme Simonin for translating the book for the French edition.

My grateful thanks go to the many B1 users who have offered their stories to add further information about the successful use of B1 for Parkinson's.

Finally, my thanks go to Duncan Swindells of *Ex Libris Digital Press* who has worked tirelessly in preparing my manuscript for publication.

About the Author

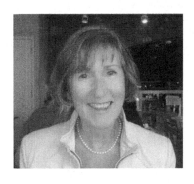

Daphne Bryan was born in Hampshire in 1948. She studied piano and voice at music college and has taught all her life. In her 50s she gained an MA and PhD in music psychology from Sheffield University. In 2010 she was diagnosed with Parkinson's and since then has researched ways to stay well. Her first book investigated how music can help Parkinson's symptoms. This second book discusses a therapy which has enabled her to continue to live a full and active life. She now lives in a village near the Trossachs in Stirlingshire, Scotland with her husband and two chickens, Winnie and Pooh.

Music as Medicine, particularly in Parkinson's

Daphne's first book was published in 2020 and is currently available on Amazon where it receives almost unanimous five-star reviews.

"This is a well-researched and very well constructed book which is both easy to read and very informative."

Made in the USA
Middletown, DE
02 March 2023